Gout

MW01534578

Kelly Bird

Apple Pie Pancakes

Minty Ginger Sweet Potato and Soup

Chicken Thyme Casserole

Avocado Cabbage Rolls

Spiced Asparagus

Morning Pie

Cinnamon Roll Bread

Avocado and Tomato Casserole

Cherry Polenta

Enchiladas Frittata

Rosemary Shells

Gout Friendly Crockpot Mac n Cheese

Marinated Eggplant

Avocado Medley

Zucchini Casserole

Thyme Stuffed Peppers

Cucumber Boats

Linguine Alfredo and Tortellini Casserole

Cornbread Casserole

Bok Choy Medley

Mini Mex Stackers

Nacho Muffins

Gout Friendly Spring Rolls

Hummus Zest

Baked Avocado Fries

Chicken Salad Celery Sticks

Meatless Stuffed Peppers

Chickpea Casserole

Chicken Teriyaki Stir-fry

Buttery Fettucine

Red Rice and Tortillas

Broccoli Curry

Risotto

Tofu Fajitas

Veggie Burger on Ciabatta With Cucumber Salad

Pot Pie Muffins

Veggie Pita

Baked Chicken Nuggets and a Chinese Veggie Salad

Greek Inspired Gout Friendly Pizza

Veggie Burger Quesadilla

Roast Beef Wraps

Honeyed Corn

Baked Tofu and Roasted Peppers

Apple Pie Cake

Baked Peppered Taquitos

5 alarm Baked Chicken Wings

Kale and Tofu:

Stuffed Pepper Melts

White Pepper Roasted Chicken

Wings and Watermelon Salad

These recipes are not intended to be any type of Medical advice. ALL individuals must consult their Doctors first and should always receive their meal plans from a qualified practitioner. . These recipes are not intended to heal, or cure anyone from any kind of illness, or disease

Apple Pie Pancakes

- 1 cup wheat flour
- 1/3 teaspoon baking powder
- ¼ teaspoon baking soda
- ¼ teaspoon cinnamon
- 1/2 teaspoon apple pie spice
- 1 teaspoon brown sugar
- ½ cup low or no fat milk**
- 1 cup crushed pecans (optional)
- 1 can low or no sugar added apple pie filling (optional)

1. Mix together flour, baking soda, and baking powder. Some sources say those on a low purine diet should limit whole grain and wheat based foods to 1-2 servings a week, if needed white flour may be substituted.

2. Stir in the cinnamon, apple pie spice, and brown sugar

3. Incorporate the milk. The dough should be pliable and easy to work with, if it is not add more milk 1 tablespoon at a time.

4. If desired mix crushed pecans into the mix

5. Before serving top the pancakes with the apple pie filling for added apple flavor!

6. Pour a fist sized (or smaller for silver dollar pancakes) onto a hot griddle and let cook until bubbles form around the edges, approx. 2-3 minutes.

7.   Flip and repeat

Nutritional Information:

- Calories: 79
- Total Fat: 7 g
- Carbohydrates: 4g
- Protein: 4g

Minty Ginger Sweet Potato and Soup

- 1 tablespoon olive oil
- 2 medium-large sweet potato peeled, chopped, and pureed
- 1 clove garlic
- 1 teaspoon ginger
- 1/3 teaspoon turmeric
- 4 diced mint leaves
- 2 cup no sodium beef or vegetable broth

1. Pour olive oil into food processor
2. Wash, peel, cut into small pieces, and place sweet potato bits into the food processor with the oil.
3. Add garlic clove to the food processor
4. Add the ginger, turmeric. Turmeric is a anti-inflammatory and has shown success in aiding gout inflammation. Chili powder or cayenne powder can be substituted though.
5. Wash, dry, and chop mint leaves. Like turmeric, mint has health benefits, however, thyme can be substituted for it.
6. Puree
7. Pour into medium sized pot or Dutch oven
8. Add broth
9. Let sit over medium-medium high heat 25-30 minutes.

10.   Best served with toasted bread.

Nutritional Info:

Calories: 140

Total Fats: 4.0 g

Carbohydrates: 26.9 g

Protein: 4.0 g

Chicken Thyme Casserole

- 1 cup boneless, skinless chicken thigh pieces, approx. 1x1
- ¾ cup brown rice
- ½ cup water
- ½ cup diced carrots
- ½ cup peas
- 2 teaspoon thyme
- 1 teaspoon celery salt
- ¼ teaspoon black pepper

1. Using a Dutch oven or large pot brown the chicken pieces
2. Pour in brown rice kernels
3. Pour in water and stir
4. Add carrots, peas, thyme, celery salt, and pepper
5. Bring to boil, reduce heat to low, cover and let simmer 20-30 minutes stirring occasionally.

Nutritional Information:

Calories: 143

Total Fat: 46.4

Carbohydrates: 34.6 mg

Protein: 16.5 g

Avocado Cabbage Rolls

- 1 tablespoon olive oil
- 1 tablespoon apple cider vinegar
- 1 large avocado diced
- 1 head of cabbage
- 1 small onion diced
- ½ tablespoon chili powder

1. Preheat oven to 425 and prepare baking tray
2. Add 1 tablespoon olive oil to hot skillet
3. Sauté onion for 1 minute
4. Add chili powder, mix well into onion
5. Mix in one tablespoon apple cider vinegar and avocado pieces
6. Sauté 30-45 seconds and remove from heat
7. Lay out cabbage leaves, fill each leaf with 1 spoonful of mix
8. Lay on prepared baking tray and cook for 12-14 minutes

Nutritional Information:

Calories: 76

Total Fat: 3.5

Carbohydrates: 31 mg

Protein: 4.6 g

Spiced Asparagus

- 10-12 asparagus spears
- 1 tablespoon of olive oil
- ½ tablespoon jalapeno powder
- 1 cup plain bread crumbs
- 1 cup parmesan cheese

1. Preheat oven to 400 and prepare a baking tray
2. Wash and dry asparagus spears and set aside
3. In a bowl mix together the olive oil, jalapeno powder, bread crumbs, and parmesan cheese
4. Using tongs or a fork roll the asparagus spears in the bowls mixture, make sure it's thoroughly covered, and lay out on the tray
5. Cook 20-23 minutes or until cheese turns golden brown

Nutrition Information:
Calories: 89
Total Fat: 3.4
Carbohydrates: 9.7 mg
Protein: 5.7 g

Morning Pie

1 tablespoon oil or spray

1 teaspoon garlic and parsley powder

1/3 cup salsa

4 egg white

1 frozen roll biscuit dough

1/2 cup cheddar or Colby jack cheese

Prepare crockpot

Add oil or spray bottom of pot

Pour in garlic & parsley powder, salsa, egg whites, and stir together

Cover with piece of biscuit dough and top it off with the cheese'

Cook 2 hours on high

Nutritional Information:

Calories: 321

Total Fat: 34

Carbohydrates: 43 mg

Protein: 13.4 g

Cinnamon Roll Bread

1 roll cinnamon rolls

2 tablespoons butter, melted

2 cups confectioners' sugar

2/3 cup lemon juice

3/4 tablespoon brown sugar

4 teaspoon cinnamon

1 cup pecan pieces

Raisins

In a small bowl mix confectioners' sugar and lemon juice stirring until you get a thin consistency. If more lemon juice is needed add 1 tsp at a time.

In another bowl mix together the brown sugar, cinnamon, and pecan pieces and set aside

Roll cinnamon dough into one flat sheet that will fit down inside your crockpot. If you need to "double-up" some edges to get it to fit that's fine.

Coat the inside of the crockpot with cooking spray

Add cinnamon roll and pour the melted butter over them.

Cook 1 hour on high

Coat with confectioners' sugar and then the brown sugar/cinnamon/ pecan mixture and cook on high another 30 minutes.

When done top with raisins.

Nutritional Information:

Calories: 456

Total Fat: 46

Carbohydrates: 46.4 mg

Protein: 15.7 g

Avocado and Tomato Casserole

Cubed or torn ciabatta bread

1 tablespoon olive oil

1/3 cup diced scallions

1/2 can diced tomatoes

1 large or 2 medium avocados diced

3 finely diced basil leaves or 1 tablespoon

1 cup mozzarella cheese

Preheat oven to 350 and prepare a 11x9 casserole dish.

In a small bowl mix together olive oil, scallions, tomatoes, avocados and basil.

Place bread into casserole dish and top with tomato/avocado mixture.

Top with mozzarella cheese

Cook uncovered 18-22 minutes.

Nutritional Information:

Calories: 87

Total Fat: 13.7

Carbohydrates: 9.2

Protein: 11.1 g

Cherry Polenta

Olive oil

1 tablespoon butter

2 cup polenta

2 cup low fat milk

1 1/2 cup cherry

Spray or wipe olive oil in large pot or Dutch oven

Add butter, polenta, and low fat milk and stir well.

Bring to a boil, reduce heat, and simmer 40-45 minutes

Stir in cherries.

Nutritional Information:

Calories: 136

Total Fat: 45

Carbohydrates: 30.9 mg

:

Proteins: 6.7 g

Enchiladas Frittata

Butter

Canola or vegetable oil

5-7 large egg whites

½ can low sodium, no salt added, petite tomatoes

1/3 cup salsa

1 teaspoon hot sauce

2/3 tablespoon chili powder

1 teaspoon cumin

1 teaspoon celery salt

1 package cheddar cheese or Mexican blend cheese

1 teaspoon cilantro (optional)

Prepare skillet or Dutch oven over medium high heat, letting butter melt and mix with the olive oil.

 Mix together egg whites, tomatoes, salsa, hot sauce, chili powder, cumin, and celery salt. Top with cheese and let set. Periodically push a spatula under it to insure that it doesn't stick.

Cook, uncovered, 18-22 minutes

Nutritional Information:

Calories: 101

Total Fat: 10.3

Carbohydrates: 34.3 mg

Protein: 9

Rosemary Shells

1 tablespoon olive oil, divided

1 package stuffed shells

1 tablespoon finely diced rosemary

½ cup ricotta cheese

1/2 cup diced tomatoes

Preheat oven to 400; pour ½ tablespoon olive oil into 9x9 casserole dish

 Lay out shells open side up

In a small bowl mix together rosemary, cheese, and tomatoes.

Spoon mixture into shells

Drizzle with olive oil

Cook 30 minutes or as directed by package.

Nutritional Information:

Calories: 78

Total Fat: 32.3

Carbohydrates: 46 mg

Protein: 14 g

Gout Friendly Crockpot Mac n Cheese

1 tablespoon vegetable oil

1 tablespoon butter

1 teaspoon garlic and parsley powder

1 teaspoon onion powder

1 tablespoon sriracha sauce

1 cup low or no sodium chicken bouillon

1/2 cup low fat milk

1 8 oz. box elbow macaroni

1 cup Monterey Jack cheese

1/2 cups plain bread crumbs

Place in the bottom of the crockpot: olive oil, butter, garlic powder and parsley, onion powder, sriracha sauce chicken bouillon, and milk

Pour in the macaroni and cheese and stir well.

Cook 1 ½ hours on low.

Thirty minutes before its done top with the bread crumbs.

Nutritional Information:

Calories: 178

Total Fat: 59

Carbohydrates 56.1 mg:

Protein: 27.4

Marinated Eggplant

1 tablespoon oil

1/2 tablespoon butter

1/3 cup honey

1 teaspoon Worcester sauce

1/3 brown sugar

1 tablespoon ginger powder or minced

1 teaspoon black pepper

1 small onion diced

1 cup diced eggplant

In plastic bag mix oil, butter, honey, brown sugar, ginger, pepper

Place eggplant and onion pieces in marinade and let sit in refrigerator 4 hours

Over oil sauté onions and eggplant over medium high heat 5 minutes.

Nutritional Information:

Calories: 111

Total Fat: 14.5

Carbohydrates: 18.7 mg

Proteins: 5.6 g

Avocado Medley

¾ tablespoon olive oil

1 cup brown rice

¾ cup water

Garlic and parsley powder

1 tomato diced

1 onion diced

1 cup eggplant diced

1 diced avocado

1/4 cup lemon juice

1 tablespoon diced basil

Pour olive oil in a Dutch oven or large pot and let warm over high heat. Sauté tomato, onion, eggplant, and avocado for 1-2 minutes.

Pour lemon juice, rice, water, and garlic and parsley powder and bring to a boil stirring frequently.

Reduce heat to low, cover, and simmer 25 minutes stirring occasionally.

Nutritional Information:

Calories: 57

Total Fat: 16

Carbohydrates: 24.9 mg

Protein: 4.8 g

Zucchini Casserole

2-3 zucchinis cubed in 2x2 pieces

1 cup mozzarella cheese

1/3 cup olive oil

1/2 tablespoon parsley

½ tablespoon rosemary

Preheat oven to 400 and prepare a 9x9 casserole dish.

Wash, dry, and cube zucchini; place in a bowl.

Pour in bowl with zucchini, cheese, oil, parsley, and rosemary

Cook 18-20 minutes.

Nutritional Information:

Calories: 77

Total Fat: 43

Carbohydrates: 39 mg

Protein: 6.4 g

Thyme Stuffed Peppers

2 bell peppers, cleaned

1 tablespoon olive oil

1/2 cup uncooked rice

1 can no salt added diced tomatoes

1 cup beef broth

1/2 tablespoon thyme

½ cup parmesan cheese

Wash, dry, cut the tops off and clean out the ribs and seeds inside the peppers.

Put them inside crockpot

In a small bowl mix together rice, tomatoes, broth, and thyme

Spoon mixture into peppers then sprinkle tops of stuffed peppers with cheese

Cook on low 3-4 hours.

Nutritional Information:

Calories: 134

Total Fat: 24

Carbohydrates: 21 mg

Protein: 12.2 g

Cucumber Boats

2 cucumbers, centers removed

1 diced tomatoes

1 diced shallot

1 tablespoon low sodium Italian dressing

1/3 cup mozzarella cheese (optional)

1/2 tablespoon chia seeds

Preheat oven to 325 and prepare baking tray.

Wash and dry the cucumbers. Cut cucumbers in half a hollow out the centers, roughly 1x2

Lay open side up on tray

In small bowl mix together tomatoes, shallot, Italian dressing, and cheese

Spoon mixture into 'trench' and top with seeds.

Cook 12-15 minutes

Nutritional Information:

Calories: 87

Total Fat: 9.4

Carbohydrates: 0.8 mg

Protein: 2.3 g

Linguine Alfredo and Tortellini Casserole

1 tablespoon olive oil

1 teaspoon minced garlic

½ shallot, diced

2 cups worth cheese tortellini

1 cup Alfredo sauce

1 teaspoon oregano

1 cup Italian blend cheese

1 8oz. box linguine

Preheat oven to 350 and prepare a 9x9 casserole dish

Cook linguine according to package directions, drain, and put back in pot and set aside ,

In skillet over med. high heat, add oil and sauté garlic and onion 2-3 minutes.

Pour sautéed onions and garlic into linguine, as well as, Alfredo sauce, tortellini, oregano, and Italian blend cheese, and stir well.

Pour into dish and bake 25-30 minutes

Nutritional Information:

Calories: 213

Total Fat: 24.6

Carbohydrates: 54.5 mg

Protein: 12 g

Cornbread Casserole

Butter, melted

2/3 cup green beans, drained

½ cup whole kernel corn

½ cup diced carrots

3 cups crumbled cornbread

1 teaspoon sage

½ teaspoon cloves

Preheat oven to 350 and prepare 9x9 casserole dish.

In a bowl mix together melted butter, beans, corn, carrots, sage, and cloves

Crumble cornbread into the bottom of the casserole dish

Spoon bean mixture on top of cornbread

Cook, uncovered, for 25-30 minutes.

Nutritional Information:

Calories: 345

Total Fat: 46.9

Carbohydrates: 56.4 mg

Protein: 24 g

Bok Choy Medley

1 cup jasmine rice

1 tablespoon apple cider vinegar

1/3 cup organic honey

½ teaspoon black pepper

½ teaspoon cayenne powder

1 finely diced bok choy

1 cup fajita peppers and onions

Preheat oven to 350 and prepare 9x9 casserole dish.

Put one cup of rice in bottom of dish; pour in apple cider vinegar and honey.

Wash, dry, and dice on stalk of bok choy.

Place bok choy, fajitas, onions, black pepper, and cayenne powder on top of rice.

Cover with foil and cook for 30 minutes.

Nutritional Information:

Calories: 101

Total Fat: 11.1

Carbohydrates: 13 mg

Proteins: 5 g

Mini Mex Stackers

10 corn tortilla shells

1/3 cup turmeric powder

2 cups salsa

1/2 can black beans drained and wash

1 package Mexican blend cheese

Preheat oven to 350 and prepare a baking tray

In a bowl mix together turmeric powder, salsa, and black beans.

Using a biscuit cutter, cut 3 inch circles out of each tortilla. You can either make numerous 1 layer pizzas or multiple multi-layer pizzas.

Lay down a piece of tortilla, add I spoonful of mixture and cover with cheese

Cook, uncovered, 15-18 minutes or until cheese is melted

Nutritional Information:

Calories: 234

Total Fat: 25.5

Carbohydrates: 43.1 mg

Protein: 3.4 g

Nacho Muffins

1 package low sodium tortilla chips

1 tablespoon vegetable oil

1 cup low sodium petite diced tomatoes

2 diced scallions

2 teaspoons chili powder

1 teaspoon chopped basil

3 oz. shredded chicken, pre-cooked (optional)

1 cup Mexican blend cheese

Prepare muffin molds and preheat oven to 350.

In food processor mix tortilla chips and vegetable oil until it is worked into a fine consistency and press into the bottom of the molds.

In another bowl mix together tomatoes, scallions, spices, and chicken if using.

Spoon into muffin molds.

Cook 28-32 minutes.

*If mix needs more oil add 1 teaspoon at a time.

Nutritional Information:

Calories: 456

Total Fat: 19.7

Carbohydrates: 46.3 mg

Protein: 23 g

Gout Friendly Spring Rolls

6-7 rice paper wrappers

1/2 cup carrot matchsticks

1/2 cup sliced cucumber

1 cup diced avocado

1 teaspoon white wine vinegar

1 teaspoon lemon juice

½ tablespoon apple cider vinegar

Preheat oven to 350 and prepare baking tray.

Layout wrappers on tray.

In a bowl mix together carrots, cucumber, avocado, vinegar, lemon juice, and apple cider vinegar

Place 1 spoonful of mixture into each wrapper and roll up

Cook 30 minutes

Nutritional Information:

Calories: 123

Total Fat: 3.2

Carbohydrates: 9 mg:

Protein: 14 g

Hummus Zest

2/3 cup low sodium chickpeas

1/2 tablespoon olive oil or coconut oil

1 teaspoon red pepper flakes

1 teaspoon chopped oregano

1/2 teaspoon thyme

Rinse chickpeas and drain

Put all chickpeas, oil, red pepper flakes, oregano, and thyme in food processor and blend.

Store in an airtight container in the refrigerator; will keep 3-5 days.

Nutritional Information:

Calories: 145

Total Fat 7.5:

Carbohydrates: 35.3 mg

Protein: 8.3 g

Baked Avocado Fries

3 egg whites

½ cup flour

1/3 cup low sodium breadcrumbs

¼ cup parmesan cheese

2 large avocado, cut into French fry shape

Preheat oven to 425 and prepare a baking tray

In a small bowl mix egg whites together

In a second bowl, mix together flour, breadcrumbs, and cheese

Dip avocado pieces into the egg mix, then the flour mix and place on baking tray roughly 1 inch apart.

Cook 20-22 minutes

Nutritional Information:

Calories: 61

Total Fat: 1.4

Carbohydrates: 9.9 mg

Protein: 4.5 g

Chicken Salad Celery Sticks

4-5 celery stalk each cut into 3 pieces

3 oz. cream cheese

1/3 teaspoon basil

¼ - 1/3 cup cooked chicken cubes

½ tablespoon chia seeds (optional)

Let cream cheese sit out and soften for 30 minutes

Wash and dry stalks; cut each stalk into 3 pieces

In a bowl mix soften cream cheese, basil, and chicken.

 Spread dip into celery centers. Dip will 3-5 days if kept in an air tight container in the refrigerator.

Nutritional Information:

Calories: 34.9

Total Fat: 6.5

Carbohydrates: 3.4 mg

Protein: 12.4 g

Meatless Stuffed Peppers

1 cup cauliflower mash (instructions below)

¾ tablespoon melted butter, or coconut oil

1/3 tablespoon minced garlic or garlic powder

4 bell peppers

1/2 cup eggplant cubed, diced

1 teaspoon basil

½ teaspoon oregano

Preheat oven to 350 and prepare 9x9 casserole dish

Wash, dry, and remove the ribs and seeds from the peppers. Put in dish when done.

In a food processor add cauliflower, oil or butter, and garlic and puree until a mashed potato consistency is achieved

Spoon mixture in peppers

Top with pieces of eggplant, basil, oregano, and cheese

Bake, covered, 25-30 minutes.

Nutritional Information:

Calories: 134

Total Fat: 24

Carbohydrates: 7.3 mg

Protein: 12.8 g

Chickpea Casserole

1 can low sodium chickpeas (garbanzo beans)

1 teaspoon olive oil

1/2 cup water

1/4 cup dry white wine or cooking white wine

2 teaspoon chili powder

1 teaspoon red pepper flakes

2 cup uncooked rice

Drain beans and wash

Put all ingredients in crockpot

Cook on high 1 hour

Nutritional Information:

Calories: 123

Total Fat: 24.3

Carbohydrates: 46vmg

Protein: 15 g

Chicken Teriyaki Stir-fry

3 oz. chicken cubes

2 teaspoon brown sugar

1 tablespoon raw organic honey

1/2 teaspoon low sodium sesame oil (optional)

1 cup cooked jasmine rice

1/2 cup bell pepper strips

1/3 cup baby corn

In plastic bag marinate chicken cubes overnight in the refrigerator in brown sugar, honey, and sesame oil.

Put chicken into wok and cook until done, add rice, peppers, and corn and warm through.

Nutritional Information:

Calories: 97

Total Fat: 14.4

Carbohydrates: 32.3 mg

Protein: 8.7 g

Buttery Fettucine

4 oz. fettucine

1/2 tablespoon melted butter

1 teaspoon chopped oregano

1 teaspoon thyme

1 teaspoon basil

Cook fettucine for 8 minutes until al dente, drain but do not rinse.

Melt butter with chopped oregano, thyme, and basil, and pour over fettucine.

Nutritional Information:

Calories: 104

Total Fat: .8

Carbohydrates: 28 mg

Protein: 7.8 g

Red Rice and Tortillas

2 cups cooked rice

3 oz. ground beef ,drained and browned

1/2 tablespoon chili powder

1/2 teaspoon cumin

2 8 or 10 inch tortilla shells (corn work best)

Olive oil or melted butter

Place rice into pot on stove, add water, protein, and spices; bring to a boil and then reduce heat to low and let simmer, stirring occasionally

Cook approx. 25-30 minutes

Place tortilla shells on top of each other and cut into 4 triangles

Spread out on a baking tray and 'paint' oil or butter on the triangles with a sauce brush. Cook at 400 approx. 20-22 minutes.

Nutritional Information:

Calories: 84

Total Fat: .8

Carbohydrates: 11 mg

Protein: 17 g

Broccoli Curry

½ tablespoon vegetable oil

2/3 cup broccoli

½ cup tofu (optional)

1 cup uncooked rice

1/2 cup water

1 tablespoon coconut milk or soy milk

1/2 tablespoon turmeric

In pot, or Dutch oven, over medium high heat, pour in oil and sauté broccoli and tofu.

Add the uncooked rice, water, coconut milk or soy milk and bring to a boil, reduce heat, and cover.

Let simmer 28-30 minutes. Stir often so rice does not stick to bottom of pot.

Nutritional Information:

Calories: 89

Total Fat: 9

Carbohydrates: 16mg

Protein: 24 g

Risotto

3 oz. lean, low sodium diced ham

1 tablespoon butter

1 tablespoon olive oil

2 cups uncooked Arborio rice

1 cup vegetable bouillon cube

1/3 teaspoon black pepper

1/4 teaspoon orange peel

2 diced scallions

In pot melt butter, pour in the olive oil and pour in uncooked rice, letting it toast while stirring it around to ensure that all sides are toasted evenly; continue this 5-7 minutes over medium-high heat.

Add ham, bullion and spices; bring to a boil, reduce heat to medium while stirring constantly.

Top with scallions before serving

Nutritional Information:

Calories: 312

Total Fat: 23.7

Carbohydrates: 54.8 mg

Protein: 6 g

Tofu Fajitas

4 corn tortilla shells, warmed

½ tablespoon butter

1 tablespoon coconut oil

1 large sweet onion, cut into strips and caramelized

2 bell peppers sliced into strips

1 block firm tofu

2 teaspoon lemon juice

1 teaspoon cayenne pepper

½ teaspoon cumin

Paint some oil on each side of the corn shell, warm shell in skillet 2-3 minutes on each side. Can keep warm if wrapped in aluminum foil and kept in 200 degree oven.

Wash, dry, and cut into strips onions, peppers, and tofu.

In large pot let oil and butter mix over med. High heat.

Add onion strip and sauté stirring until a brown-gold and very fragrant, approx. 2-3 minutes. Add peppers and tofu and cook approx. 1 minute. Remove and drain

Nutritional Information:

Calories: 211

Total Fat: 16.7

Carbohydrates: 48.5 mg

Protein: 23 g

Veggie Burger on Ciabatta With Cucumber Salad

1 low sodium ciabatta roll

1 veggie burger (4 oz. preferably soy-based)

1 teaspoon brown sugar

1 teaspoon thyme leaves

1 onion 1/4 of it cut into rounds

1 cucumber

4 cherry tomatoes

1 shallot

1/3 cup olive oil

1 tablespoon white wine vinegar

½ tablespoon basil

Wash vegetables thoroughly even if labeled organic.

Cut cucumbers in half-moon shapes; cut cherry tomatoes into halves and cut them in half cut the onions in strips .

Put pieces into a bowl and add olive oil, vinegar, and basil. Cover and store in Refrigerator until ready to eat.

In a small bowl brown sugar and thyme and sprinkle onto uncooked veggie burger. Cook burger according to directions, seasonings will not affect cooking time.

Nutritional Information:

Calories: 217 mg

Total Fat: 7.6 mg

Carbohydrates: 41 mg

Protein: 31 g

Pot Pie Muffins

1 package phylo dough

3 oz. boneless skinless chicken breast, cooked and shredded (optional)

1 cup cauliflower

½ cup chicken bouillon

1/3 cup low sodium vegetable mix (carrots, corn, beans, peas, etc.)

1 teaspoon garlic and parsley seasoning

1/8 teaspoon sage

Prepare muffin molds and preheat oven to 375.

Wash and dry cauliflower and place in food processor along with chicken bouillon. Mix until a consistency like mashed potatoes is reached.

In a bowl mix together chicken, mash, and seasonings.

Lay dough on floured flat surface and cut dough into to circles to fit inside muffin holes. Use an upside down cup to help with this.

Fill each muffin with half a spoonful of mixture and cover with the edges of dough circle. Pierce top with fork a few times or create 1 inch slits to allow steam to escape.

Cook 18-22 minutes.

Nutritional Information:

Calories: 321 mg

Total Fat: 14.7 mg

Carbohydrates: 57.6 mg

Protein: 21.6 g

Veggie Pita

1 small, low sodium, pita pocket halved

1 teaspoon smoky paprika

1/4 teaspoon black pepper

1/3 cup diced bok choy pieces

1/3 cup diced avocado pieces

1/3 cup diced cucumber pieces

1/3 cup matchstick carrots

1/3 cup diced cherry tomatoes

1 teaspoon lemon juice

Turn on broiler onto high and prepare baking tray

Wash, dry, and dice all vegetables.

Put vegetables into a bowl, add spices, and lemon juice; mix well.

Spoon mix inside pita's and warm in broiler 2-4 minutes.

Nutritional Information:

Calories: 312

Total Fat: 23mg

Carbohydrates: 68mg

Protein: 12g

Baked Chicken Nuggets and a Chinese Veggie Salad

3 oz. boneless skinless chicken breast or thighs, cubed 2x2

2 egg whites

Salt free breadcrumbs

No-salt herb seasoning

1-2 cup Chinese cabbage

1 stalk chopped bok choy

3 oz. beansprouts

Prepare baking tray with parchment paper or aluminum foil, and preheat oven to 375.

In one bowl scramble egg mixture, in second mix together breadcrumbs and seasoning

Dredge chicken through egg coating and then through the breadcrumbs, taking care to coat both sides.

Lay 2 inches apart on tray and cook 22-27 minutes.*Under cooked chicken can be hazardous to your health so be sure to cut into a piece checking for any running juices or pink meat before consuming. A longer cooking time or higher oven temp might be needed.

Wash and dry

In a bowl toss together cabbage, bok choy, and beansprouts

Nutritional Information:

Calories: 562

Total Fat: 27.8

Carbohydrates: 119 mg

Protein: 32.1 g

Greek Inspired Gout Friendly Pizza

2 tablespoon olive oil

1 cup Feta cheese crumbled

4 cup cherry tomatoes, halved and halved again

1 cup radish, diced

1 cup avocado, diced

1/3 cup diced low sodium black olives (optional)

1 teaspoon red pepper flakes

1 tablespoon coarsely chopped basil leaves

1 teaspoon diced oregano

1 low sodium or no sodium small pizza shell, pizza dough, or flatbread

Lay out dough and using a sauce brush 'paint' with olive oil

Sprinkle with seasoning and cheese

Add remaining ingredients.

Bake according to shell/dough instructions.

Nutritional Information:

Calories: 224

Total Fat: 7.2

Carbohydrates: 45 mg

Protein: 13.5 g

Veggie Burger Quesadilla

2 10 inch burrito tortilla

3 oz. veggie burger crumbled

1/4 cup cheddar cheese or Mexican blend

1/3-1/2 cup scallions, 1-2 diced

1 teaspoons chili powder

1/2 teaspoon cumin

1 teaspoon diced cilantro

Or 1 tablespoon Mrs. Dash Mexican seasoning in lieu of chili powder and cumin

Spray skillet with no-stick cooking spray, preheat over high heat, and turn heat down to med.-high before cooking.

Layer ingredients on 1 tortilla shell, make sure the cheese goes on top as it acts like a glue to hold the other shell on

Lay the other tortilla shell on top when done

To make flipping easier cut into pieces with a pizza cutter.

Cook approx. 3-4 minutes on each side

Nutritional Information:

Calories: 134

Total Fat: 5.6

Carbohydrates: 47 mg

Protein: 18 g

Roast Beef Wraps

1 sandwich wrap

Two slices but no more than 3 oz. Roast Beef,

1 tablespoon lite onion dip powder

1 roasted pepper sliced into strips

1 tomato cut into thick slices roasted

1 oz. sliced mushrooms (optional)

1 oz. spinach (optional)

1 tablespoon apple cider vinegar

1 teaspoon lemon juice

1 dash pepper or red pepper flakes

Wash, dry, and prepare all vegetables.

Layout wrap

In small bowl mix together onion dip powder, veggie slices, mushrooms, spinach, apple cider vinegar, lemon juice, and red pepper flakes.

Lay roast beef down on wrap, spoon mixture on top, roll up wrap and enjoy.

Nutritional Information:

Calories: 112

Total Fat: 0.4 mg

Carbohydrates: 21 mg

Protein: 11 g

Honeyed Corn

4 ears of corn

1 tablespoon of melted butter

3 tablespoon of organic honey

2/3 tablespoon apple cider vinegar

1 tablespoon turmeric

In a small bowl mix together melted butter, honey, vinegar, and turmeric.

With a sauce brush thoroughly coat each ear of corn.

Wrap in foil and cook on grill over medium flame 20-25 minutes

Nutritional Information:

Calories: 38

Total Fat: 16

Carbohydrates: 43

Protein: 6 g

Baked Tofu and Roasted Peppers

Olive oil

1/2 shallot diced

1/2 container firm tofu, cubed and dried

1/3 cup water

1 tablespoon dry white wine or white cooking wine

1 teaspoon red pepper slices

Preheat oven to 400 and prepare a 9x9 casserole dish

Wash, dry, and prepare shallots, tofu, and peppers for baking

Pour ingredients into dish

Cook 20-25 minutes.

Nutritional Information:

Calories: 56

Total Fat: 9 mg

Carbohydrates: 14 mg

Protein: 8 g

Apple Pie Cake

1 vanilla angel food cake mix

3 large cooking apples diced

1 tablespoon honey

1 teaspoon lemon juice

½ tablespoon apple pie spice

1 teaspoon cinnamon

Spray crockpot with non-stick cooking spray

Using fat free, soy, or almond milk mix cake; pour half in the bottom of crockpot

In separate bowl mix together apples, honey, lemon juice, apple pie spice, and cinnamon

Pour apple mixture evenly on top of cake mix and pour remaining cake mix over apples

Bake 2-3 hours on low and 1-2 hours on high

Nutritional Information:

Calories: 78

Total Fat: 13

Carbohydrates: 24 mg

Protein: 4 g

Baked Peppered Taquitos

6 corn tortillas

3 oz. lean pork or chicken

1/3 cup Monterey jack cheese

1 cup no sodium diced tomatoes

1 bell pepper or jalapeno pepper

1 teaspoon chili powder

1/3 teaspoon cumin

1/2 teaspoon celery salt or celery flakes

Olive oil

Use leftovers or bake pork or chicken for 1 hour; let sit for 11-12 minutes and shred.

Preheat oven to 350 and prepare a baking tray

Use leftovers or bake pork or chicken for 1 hour; let sit for 11-12 minutes and shred.

Lay tortillas flat on baking tray

In a bowl mix together protein, cheese, tomatoes, peppers, spices

Spoon mix up and down the center of each tortilla. Keep in mind, the less filling the easier they are to roll

Roll and using a sauce brush 'paint' with olive oil

Bake in 350 degree oven 25-30 minutes

Nutritional Information:

Calories: 98

Total Fat: 43 mg

Carbohydrates: 41 mg

Protein: 34 g

5 alarm Baked Chicken Wings

3 oz. chicken wings or drumets

1 cup molasses

1/2 cup ketchup

1 tablespoon low sodium spicy mustard or wasabi

½ tablespoon organic honey

2-3 tablespoon tabasco or sriracha sauce

3 teaspoon cayenne power

1 diced jalapeno pepper

In sauce pan combine molasses, ketchup, mustard, honey, sriracha, and spices; stir, bring to a boil, and let simmer for 35 minutes

Coat the inside of the crockpot with non-stick cooking spray.

Clean and dry wings then put into crockpot and pour sauce over them. With tongs or large spoon move wings around, ensuring all are coated

If there is leftover sauce it can be stored in air tight container in refrigerator and will keep 3-5 days

Bake on high 2-2.5 hours

Nutritional Information:

Calories: 103

Total Fat: 23 mg

Carbohydrates: 26 mg

Protein: 14 g

Kale and Tofu

3oz. fresh kale leaves

3 oz. firm tofu cubes

Olive oil for drizzling

No-salt seasoning

Prepare baking tray and preheat oven to 400.

Layout individual kale leaves, drop one tofu cube in the center.

Fold leaf ends over tofu cube and flip.

Drizzle with olive oil and seasoning

 Bake 18-22 minutes.

Nutritional Information:

Calories: 17

Total Fat: 12 mg

Carbohydrates: 16mg

Protein: 9 g

Stuffed Pepper Melts

1 tablespoon of coconut oil

4 bell peppers, cleaned and hollowed

1 cup cauliflower rice

1 caramelized scallions

1 tablespoon diced mushrooms, button is fine

1 diced habanero or jalapeno pepper

1 cup feta crumbled or Monterrey jack cheese

Prepare a 9x9 baking dish and preheat the oven to 325

In a large mixing bowl mix together all ingredients, except the cheese, and spoon into hollowed out peppers.

Top with cheese, place in dish and cook, uncovered, 20-25 minutes.

Nutritional Information:

Calories: 107

Total Fat: 12.7 mg

Carbohydrates: 36mg

Protein: 12 g

White Pepper Roasted Chicken

1, 3-5 pound chicken roaster

1/3 cup olive oil

1/2 tablespoon sage

1 teaspoon orange peel

1 teaspoon rosemary

1 teaspoon white pepper

Place chicken in roasting dish and preheat the oven to 350. In a medium sized bowl mix together the oil, sage, orange peel, rosemary, pepper; cook for 1 hr. 30 minutes. .*Under cooked chicken can be hazardous to your health so be sure to cut into a piece checking for any running juices or pink meat before consuming. A longer cooking time or higher oven temp might be needed.

Nutritional Information:

Calories: 207

Total Fat: 32.7 mg

Carbohydrates: 56 mg

Protein: 58 g

Wings and Watermelon Salad

1 family package wings or drumets

1/2 watermelon, cut into 2x2 chucks

1/2 cup avocado cubes

2 cup arugula leaves

1 cup cucumber cubes

1 cup onion strips

1 cup sliced strawberries

Juice of 2 lemon

Olive oil

Sauce:

2 tablespoon paprika

1 tablespoon brown sugar

1 teaspoon cayenne powder

1 teaspoon cumin

1/4 teaspoon cinnamon

1/2 cup molasses

1 teaspoon vanilla

1/2 cup apple cider vinegar

1/3 cup ketchup

1 tablespoon mustard

Wash, dry, and prepare all ingredients.

In a bowl mix together watermelon chunks, avocado cubes, arugula leaves, cucumber leaves, strawberries, lemon juice, and cover.

Refrigerate until ready to eat

Place the wings over medium heat on your grill and with a sauce brush coat with olive oil, let cook 30 minutes

Coat all wings with sauce

Let cook 20 minutes and re-sauce.

Let cook a total of one hour; remove to foil lined container and cover them.

Nutritional Information:

Calories: 178

Total Fat: 22.3 mg

Carbohydrates: .6 mg

Protein: 34 g

As a sufferer of gout, these recipes, along with a healthy lifestyle, has really aided in controlling my flare ups. These recipes are not created to cure gout. They only are recipes that I use, and would like to share with others who may have gout, as do I. Wishing the best to you, and hope you get yours under control.

Kelly

These recipes are not intended to be any type of Medical advice. ALL individuals must consult their Doctors first and should always receive their meal plans from a qualified practitioner. . These recipes are not intended to heal, or cure anyone from any kind of illness, or disease.

Some Free Information on gout, that everyone should know, and also share with others.

GOUT

A disease that affects 1 in 100 people, over 1% of the world's total population, which was first diagnosed as early as 2640 BC is most commonly known as Gout.1, 2 Historically, Gout was referred to with a variety of other names depending on the body part in which it was located such as Podagra (foot), Gonagra (knees) and Chiagra (hands). 3   Due to links to individuals with a rich diet and excessive alcohol use, Gout has also been nick-named as the "disease of kings". 4 Hippocrates, a Greek physician known as the father of Western medicine, coined Gout with the phrase of "the unwalkable disease" in the fifth century BC. 2, 5

So, you may be asking yourself, what is Gout? Plain and simple, it is an inflammatory arthritis which is considered to be one of the most painful forms currently known to mankind. The often sudden and painful inflammation is caused by needle-like crystals that form in joints and/ or soft tissues around the joints as a result of excessive buildup of uric acid. 6 An excess of uric acid takes place when there is an increase in the normal production levels of the breakdown of purines or when the body does not eliminate enough of the acid through the kidneys in the form of urine. 7 When this occurs a condition called hyperuricemia develops in the blood which can cause an excess of uric acid crystals to form thus potentially causing Gout to develop. 7

When a person has elevated levels of uric acid and there are no other symptoms presented, it is known as Asymptomatic Gout. This is possibly the first of the four stages of Gout; however, it does not usually require any form of treatment.

The next stage is known as Acute Gout and usually leads to sudden swollen joints and intense pain resulting from the formation of the uric acid crystals described previously. The most common time this phase occurs is at night and may be linked to the use of alcohol or drugs, experiencing a period of intense stress or suffering from another illness. Whether or not treatment is administered throughout this phase, the inflammatory attack can last anywhere from a few days to nearly two weeks.

The period of time after an incidence of Acute Gout occurs is known as Intercritical Gout. During this phase there are not any symptoms. Another episode of Acute Gout may not occur for several months or years, but with each attack they can last a longer period of time and take place more often.

The last of the four phases of this disease is known as Chronic Tophaceous Gout and it is considered to be the most disabling stage. Most people do not progress to this stage if they have received proper medical treatment. Those that do enter into this stage may experience permanent damage to their kidneys and / or joints from the long term effects of this disease over the course of 10 or more years.8

With nearly 73 million people worldwide affected by Gout, who is most at risk? Those with a family history of the disease are definitely susceptible to it; however, estimates range from 20% - 80% of those with the disease have another member of their family that suffered from the disease. That is a very wide range so we need to gain a clearer understanding beyond genetics to answer this question. Individuals that are most at risk include those that are overweight, drink excessive amounts of alcohol, consume significant foods that are rich in purines, have been exposed environmentally to lead, have certain medical conditions or those that take certain medications. Additionally, men between 40 and 50 years of age and adults over 20 are more at risk than pre-menopausal women and children respectively.9

The most common medical conditions included in the at-risk list are individuals with renal insufficiencies, high blood pressure, underactive thyroid glands, psoriasis, anemia and some cancers. Kelley-Seegmiller Syndrome and Lesch-Nyhan Syndrome are two rare medical conditions that are also included on the most at risk listing.9

Medications such as diuretics, salicylate-containing drugs such as aspirin, Niacin, Cyclosporine and Levodopa which is used to treat Parkinson's disease are known to increase the risk of both hyperuricemia and gout.9

All of the cells within a person's body contain the natural substance known as purines. Additionally, purines provide a portion of the chemical structure of all plant and animal genes which means that virtually all foods will contain them.10 Those individuals that have been diagnosed with any phase of gout could benefit by avoiding excessive amounts of alcohol and reducing the consumption of foods with high concentrations of purines to help in minimizing future occurrences and symptoms. It is important to acknowledge that diet alone will not prevent or cause gout.

According to the Mayo Clinic the foods that a gout sufferer should eat and avoid are very similar to the recommendations made for anyone to have a healthy and balanced diet. Some of those recommendations include eating more fruits, vegetables and whole grains while avoiding white bread, cakes, candy, sugar-sweetened beverages and products with high-fructose corn syrup. Drinking eight to sixteen 8-ounce glasses of fluids per day with at least half of it being water keeps a person hydrated and has been known to reduce the number of gout attacks. Reducing red meats, fatty poultry and high-fat dairy products in turn reduces the intake of saturated fats. Additionally, it is also recommended to eat no more than four to six ounces of proteins from lean meat, fish and poultry and adding additional proteins from low-fat or fat-free dairy products.11

Although vegetables such as asparagus, spinach, peas, cauliflower and mushrooms contain highly concentrated levels of purines, studies have shown that they do not increase the risk of gout or increasing the number of gout attacks. Likewise, beans or lentils have moderately high levels of purines but they are a great source of protein and thus do not need to be avoided.

Supplements to your daily routine such as adding 500-mg of Vitamin C, consuming a moderate amount of regular caffeinated coffee and eating cherries has been known to help reduce the risk of gout attacks and / or reduce uric acid levels within one's body. Prior to taking Vitamin C supplements or drinking coffee should be discussed with a doctor because with certain medical conditions these items may cause other issues or interfere with other medications being taken by the patient.

Those individuals that are in the at-risk group for hyperuricemia and gout or have been diagnosed with one of the phases of gout should avoid organ and glandular meats, red meats, meat extracts, certain types of seafood and yeast products. Examples of organ and glandular meats include liver and kidney. Beef, pork and lamb are examples of red meats to avoid. Meat based soup, broth and gravy are considered meat extracts while beer and baked goods are examples of yeast products. Anchovies, sardines, herring, fish roe, canned tuna fish, shrimp, lobster, scallops and mussels are seafood that contains high levels of purine.

Some of the medications that a physician may prescribe to avoid gout flare-ups may include febuxostat (Uloric), allopurinol (Aloprim, Lopurin, Zyloprim), colchicine (Colcrys) or probenecid (Probalan). According to WebMD, it is very important that a patient taking any of these medications understands that in the first few months of beginning them that a gout attack may still flare-up. Flare-ups may still happen as a result of the patient's body is adjusting to being on the medication and does not mean that the medication does not work. The physician will likely prescribe a specific medicine for these flare-ups to take when they occur in addition to the preventative medication. Adjustments may need to be made with the dosage of the preventative medication in the event that attacks begin occurring after a long period of time taking it.12

In order to gain some symptom relief there are some non-medication pain relief remedies. For example, applying cold packs or compresses for 20 – 30 minutes several times a day to the joint affected can lessen the inflammation and help ease the pain. Elevating the affected joint on a pillow and resting will also help in reducing the pain. Again, drinking water will help in stabilizing the uric acid level to a normal level.

There are several natural remedies for treating gout at home. These include organic apple cider vinegar, baking soda, cherries, bromelain, beet juice and exercise.13

The organic apple cider vinegar is known to provide up to 90% pain relief within one to two days. To use this method of pain relief, mix one to two tablespoons of the vinegar with eight ounces of water. Once mixed, it can be drank all at once or sipped over a period of time. It is recommended to try both methods and to determine which method is most effective.

Another option for pain relief involves using the baking soda. To do so, mix eight ounces of water and mix it with one-half of a teaspoon of baking soda. It is important to drink this in one sitting; however, one may need to drink up to six glasses per day for one to two days before pain relief occurs. In some cases the first glass of the mixture may provide immediate pain relief. It is important to note that baking soda may increase blood pressure so this method may not be a good remedy for those that suffer from hypertension.

As discussed earlier, consumption of cherries can reduce the levels of uric acid in the body. A study confirmed that eating ten to twelve cherries a day reduced gout attacks by 35% and consuming up to three servings over two days reduced them by 50%.

Bromelain is a mix of a number of different protein digesting enzymes. Further, it is a natural blood thinner and anti-inflammatory that also promotes blood circulation by blocking the production of compounds that cause swelling and pain. In 1957, Ralph Heinicke, a Dole Pineapple Company chemist, discovered that pineapple stems contained high levels of this natural remedy. Pineapples are the only known fruit to contain Bromelain. Since the Bromelain is found in the stem of the pineapple it is important to take it in the form of a capsule, tablet or powder rather than just eating the fruit itself. Throughout a gout attack, take 500mg of this capsule every three hours to aid in the breakdown of the crystal-like deposits causing the attack. In order to prevent future attacks, take the same dosage twice a day on an empty stomach along with 500mg of quercentin.14

According to the Centers for disease Control and Prevention, adults should exercise for at least 30 minutes per day at a moderate intensity level most days throughout the week. This regime is known to help with the prevention of gout and also helps in reducing the intensity of the attacks. It is important to note that the exercise should not be performed during an attack. Once an attack has passed, the exercise regimen should be started back up slowly.15

For those suffering from gout it is important that their loved ones and caregivers have a good understand of the disease, the things that can prevent recurrences and the things that can help ease the symptoms during an attack. Once the knowledge about gout has been gained, the partner can be helpful by watching what the gout sufferer eats and drinks. By participating in this manner, the partner may be able to help identify the items that trigger the attacks. Additionally, the caregiver should help with reminding and encouraging their partner to continue to take medication and see their physician even after symptoms have subsided. Helping the patient get around during a flare-up and be as comfortable as possible is also extremely important since gout can be very debilitating.16

Joining a gout support group can be very helpful to those suffering from this disease and their caregivers. Some examples of these support groups are as follows:

- DailyStrength (www.dailystrength.org/c/gout/support-group)
- MDJunciton (www.mdjunction.com/gout)
- eHealth Forum (http://ehealthforum.com/health/gout.html)
- GoutPal (www.gout-pal.com/gout-pal-forum/gouty/please-help-my-gout/)
- WebMD Osteoarthritis Community (http://forums.webmd.com/3/osteoarthritis-exchange/forum/1361)

Participating in clinical trials may be another great way for a gout sufferer to help medical professionals continue to find new ways to treat and prevent the disease. There are clinical trials that are essential for pharmaceutical companies to gain FDA approval for drug use and there are clinical trials available through other organizations that do not involve drugs at all. Searching to find the right clinical trial for you can be done by visiting www.centerwatch.com. Center Watch does not perform any studies themselves but they are a publishing company that lists clinical research opportunities. It began in 1994 as a means to assist patients in finding and volunteering for such trials and to help sponsors recruit patients for the studies. Some of the trials pay patients to participate in them and others do not.

1 *The New York Times, Gout, In-Depth Report,*
  http://www.nytimes.com/health/guides/diseasses/gout-chronic/print.html

2 *US National Library of Medicine National Institutes of Health,*
  A concise history of gout and hyperuricemia and their treatment,
  http://www.ncbi.nlm.nih.gov/pubmed/16820040

3 A history of Gout (part 1). From the B.C. centuries to the end of the 19th Century AD,

  http://www.best-gout-remedies.com/historyofgout.html

4 The Sacramento Bee, Gout, the 'disease of kings', now an ailment of the masses,

  November 25, 2014, Sammy Caiola,

  http://www.sacbee.com/entertainment/living/health-fitness/article4144928.html

5   Wikipedia,   Hippocrates,
https://en.wikipedia.org/wiki/Hippocrates

6 National Institute of Arthritis and Musculoskeletal and Skin Diseases, Gout,

  http://www.niams.nih.gov/Health_Info/Gout/

7 National Institute of Arthritis and Musculoskeletal and Skin Diseases,

  What   is   Uric   Acid?,
http://www.niams.nih.gov/Health_Info/Gout/#acid

8 National Institute of Arthritis and Musculoskeletal and Skin Diseases,

  What Are the Four Stages of Gout?,

http://www.niams.nih.gov/Health_Info/Gout/#stages

9 National Institute of Arthritis and Musculoskeletal and Skin Diseases,

What Are the Four Stages of Gout?,

http://www.niams.nih.gov/Health_Info/Gout/#cause

10 The George Mateljan Foundation,

What Are Purines and in Which Foods Are They Found?

http://www.whfoods.com/genpage.php?tname=george&dbid=51

11 The Mayo Clinic, Gout diet: What's allowed, what's not,
http://www.mayoclinic.org/healthy-lifestyle/nutrition-and-healthy-eating/in-depth/gout-diet/art-20048524

12 WebMD, Treating Gout Attacks at Home,
http://www.webmd.com/arthritis/gout-attacks-at-home?page=2

13 Natural Society, Home Remedies For Gout – 12 Natural Solutions,
http://naturalsociety.com/home-remedies-for-gout-natural-solutions/

14 Spiro Koulouris Gout Blog, What is bromelain exactly and how does it help with my

gout?, http://goutandyou.com/pineapple-bromelain-and-gout/

15 Gout & Uric Acid Education Society, Gout Lifestyle Changes,

http://gouteducation.org/patient/gout-treatment/lifestyle-changes/

16 Everyday Health, Gout Attack – Role of the Caregiver,

http://www.everydayhealth.com/gout/gout-attack-role-of-the-caregiver.aspx

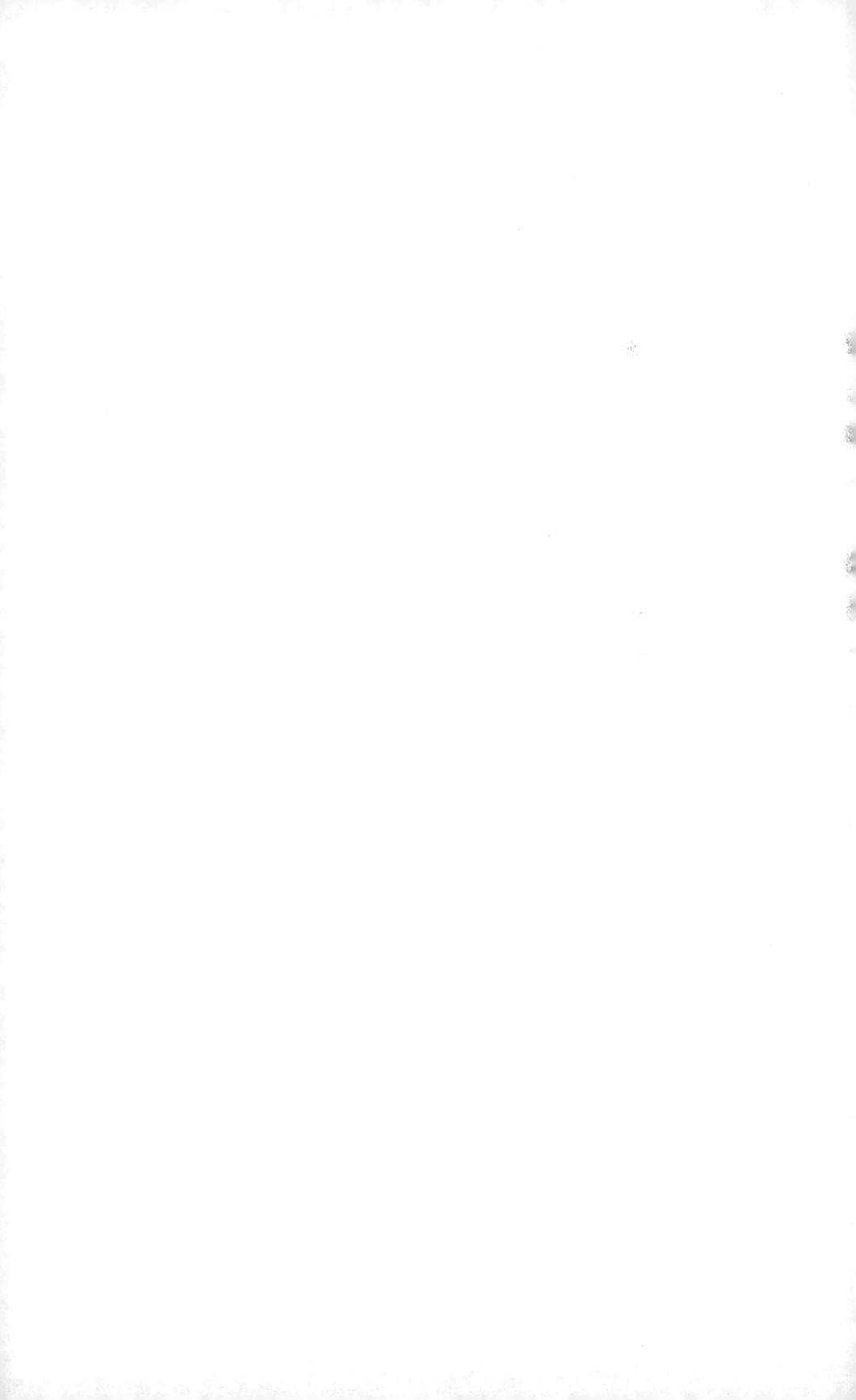

39785918R00046

Made in the USA
Middletown, DE
25 January 2017